SAY:
Synergistic Autonomy Yoga

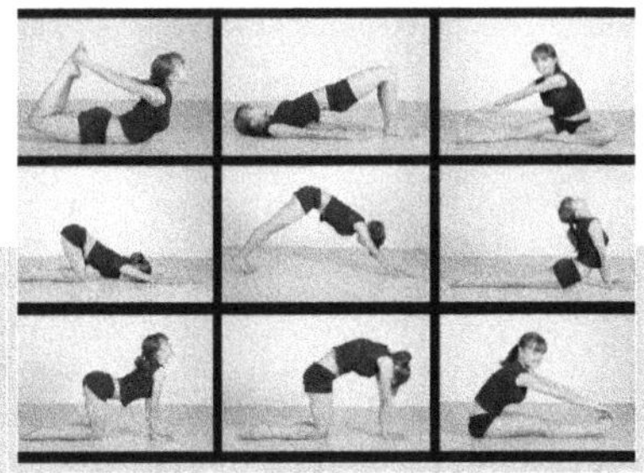

Daily Practice Manual

SAY

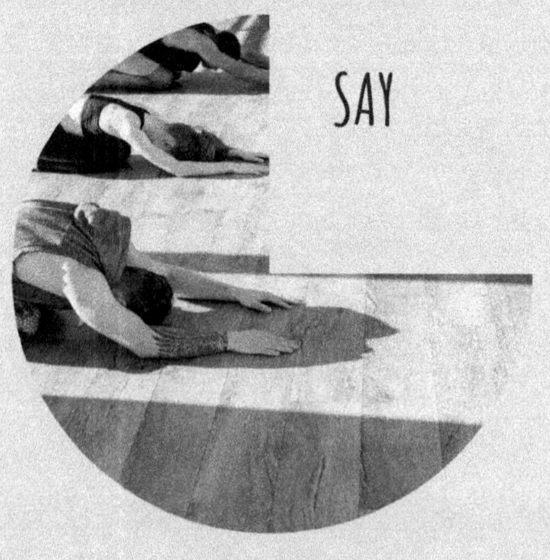

Synergistic Autonomy Yoga (SAY) is a holistic daily practice designed to integrate yoga, mindfulness, and healthy living into a balanced lifestyle. The practice emphasizes the synergy between mind and body, promoting autonomy in individual routines while fostering connectedness with others.

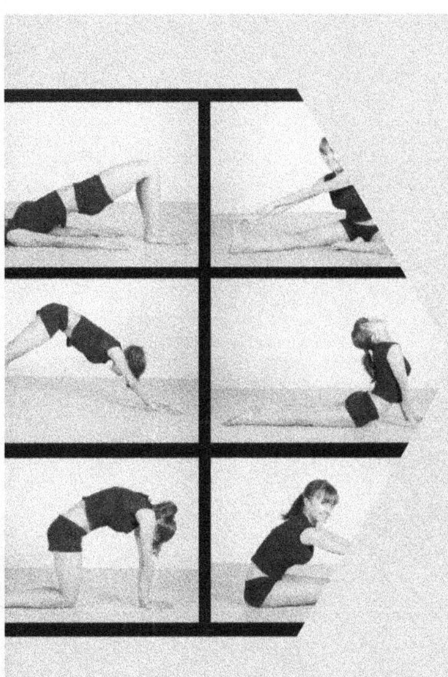

Morning Yin Flow

Morning Wake-Up Routine

1. Wake Up and Stretch:
- As you wake, gently stretch your arms and legs.
- Sit up slowly and place your feet on the floor.
- Take a moment to feel the ground beneath you.

2. Morning Thankfulness:
- Sit comfortably, close your eyes, and take three deep breaths.
- Reflect on three things you are thankful for.
- Let this gratitude fill you with a sense of peace and positivity.

3. Cleansing Breaths:
- Stand up straight, with feet hip-width apart.
- Inhale deeply through your nose, filling your lungs completely.
- Exhale slowly through your mouth, letting go of any tension.
- Repeat 5-7 times, focusing on the sensation of the breath.

4. Yin Yoga with Coffee or Tea:
- Prepare a cup of coffee and sit in a comfortable position.
- Sip your coffee mindfully, savoring each sip.
- Perform gentle yin yoga poses such as Butterfly Pose, Child's Pose, and Reclining Twist.
- Hold each pose for 3-5 minutes, focusing on deep, calming breaths.

5. Mindful Awareness Reflection with Spouse:
- Sit with your spouse and share your thoughts on the morning.
- Reflect on how you feel and your intentions for the day.
- Listen actively to each other, fostering connection and understanding.

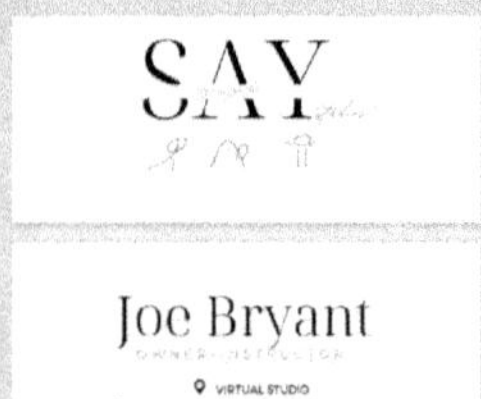

Wake-up and Stretch

Importance: Stretching upon waking helps to increase blood flow and loosen stiff muscles, setting a positive tone for the day ahead .

Meaning: This simple act signifies the beginning of a new day and prepares the body for movement.

Practical Application: As you wake, gently stretch your arms and legs while still in bed. Sit up slowly, place your feet on the floor, and stretch upward, feeling the stretch in your spine and arms.

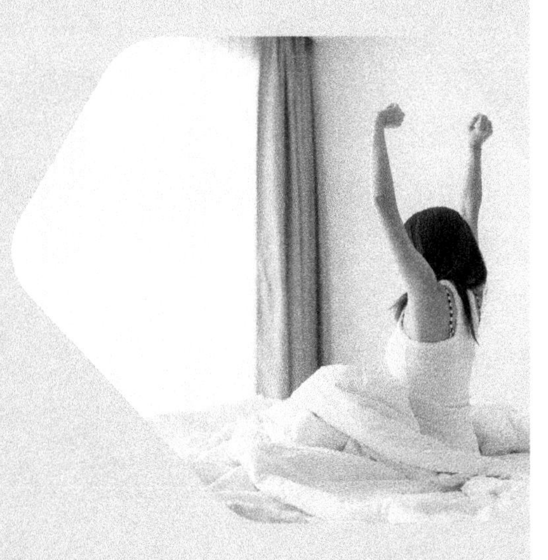

Morning Thankfulness

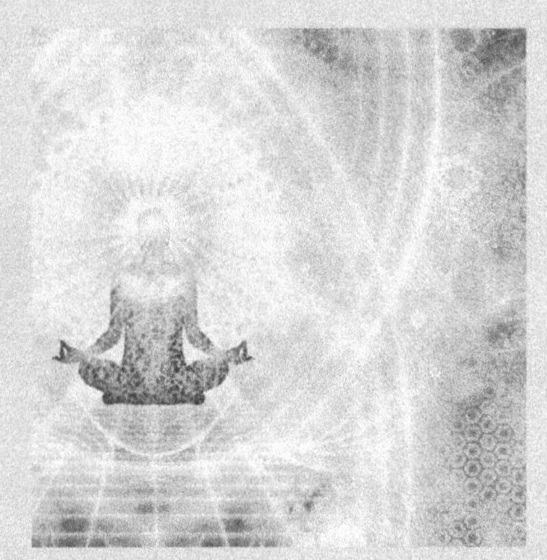

Importance: Practicing gratitude can enhance overall well-being and increase happiness .

Meaning: Reflecting on what we are thankful for can create a positive mindset, fostering resilience and joy.

Practical Application: Sit comfortably, close your eyes, and take three deep breaths. Reflect on three things you are thankful for, whether big or small. Let this gratitude fill you with a sense of peace and positivity.

Cleansing Breaths

Importance: Deep breathing exercises can reduce stress, improve mental clarity, and promote relaxation .

Meaning: These breaths cleanse the body and mind, creating a sense of calm and readiness for the day.

Practical Application: Stand up straight, with feet hip-width apart. Inhale deeply through your nose, filling your lungs completely. Exhale slowly through your mouth, letting go of any tension. Repeat 5-7 times, focusing on the sensation of the breath.

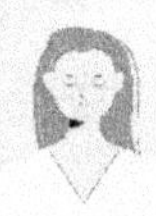

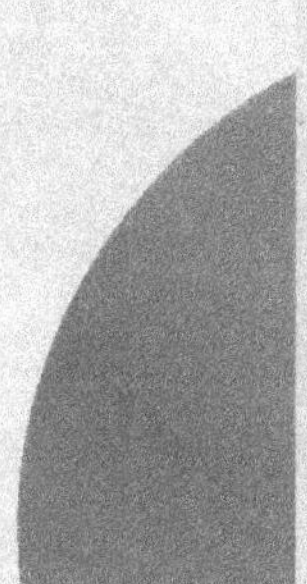

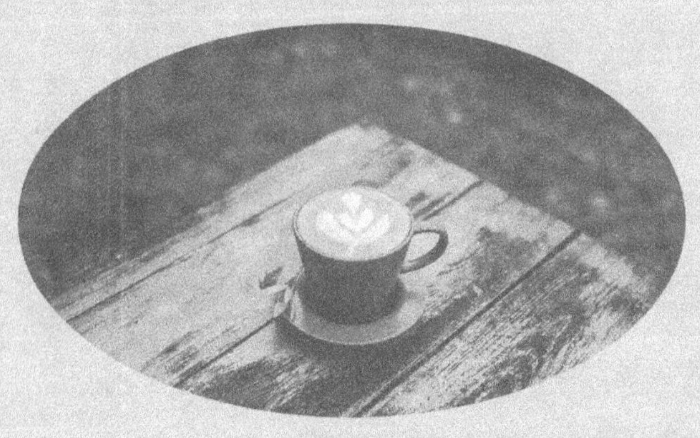

Yin YOGA with COFFEE or Tea

Importance: Combining the mindfulness of yoga with the ritual of drinking coffee or tea can enhance focus and presence .

Meaning: This routine merges physical relaxation with mindful awareness, fostering a calm yet alert state of mind.

Practical Application: Prepare a cup of coffee or tea and sit in a comfortable position. Sip your coffee mindfully, savoring each sip. Perform gentle yin yoga poses such as Butterfly Pose, Child's Pose, and Reclining Twist. Hold each pose for 3-5 minutes, focusing on deep, calming breaths.

Mindful Awareness Reflection with Spouse

Importance: Sharing thoughts and intentions with a partner can strengthen relationships and improve emotional well-being .
Meaning: This practice nurtures connection and understanding, creating a supportive start to the day.
Practical Application: Sit with your spouse and share your thoughts on the morning. Reflect on how you feel and your intentions for the day. Listen actively to each other, fostering connection and understanding.

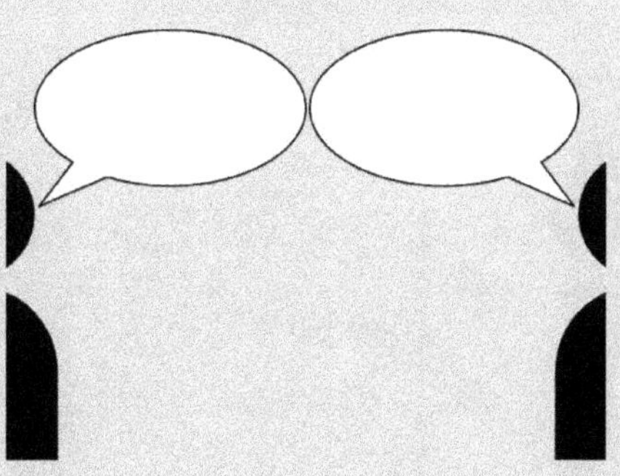

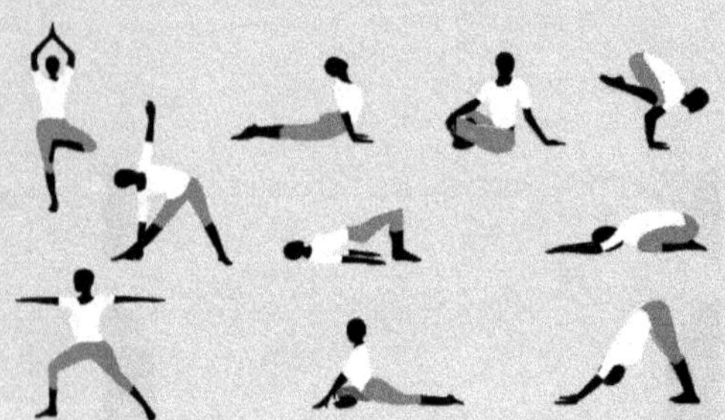

Mid-Morning Yang Yoga Practice

Synergistic Autonomy Yoga

Mid-Morning Yang Yoga Practice

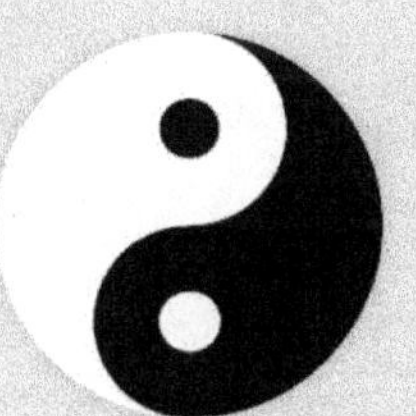

1. Indoor or Outdoor Practice:

- Choose your practice location based on the weather.
- Ensure the space is comfortable and free from distractions.

2. Vinyasa Flow:

- Begin with Sun Salutations to warm up.
- Move into a dynamic vinyasa sequence incorporating poses such as Warrior I, II, III, Downward Dog, and Plank.
- Flow continuously, linking breath with movement.

3. Dynamic Practices:

- Incorporate basketball drills or a short run to elevate your heart rate.
- Use these activities as a form of moving meditation, focusing on your breath and the rhythm of your movements.

Indoor or Outdoor Practice:

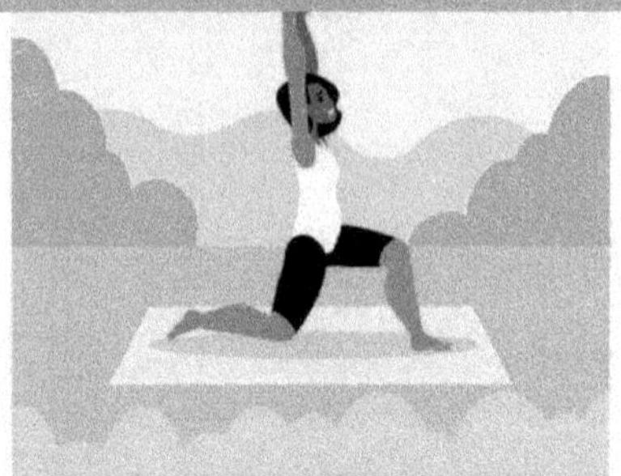

Importance: The environment can significantly impact the effectiveness of a yoga practice, with natural settings often enhancing relaxation and focus.

Meaning: Adapting the practice location based on weather encourages flexibility and mindfulness in daily routines.

Practical Application: Choose your practice location based on the weather. Ensure the space is comfortable and free from distractions. If outside, find a quiet spot with fresh air; if inside, create a calm environment with minimal interruptions.

Vinyasa Flow

Importance: Vinyasa yoga improves cardiovascular health, builds strength, and enhances flexibility .

Meaning: This dynamic flow connects breath with movement, energizing the body and mind.

Practical Application: Begin with Sun Salutations to warm up. Move into a dynamic vinyasa sequence incorporating poses such as Warrior I, II, III, Downward Dog, and Plank. Flow continuously, linking breath with movement.

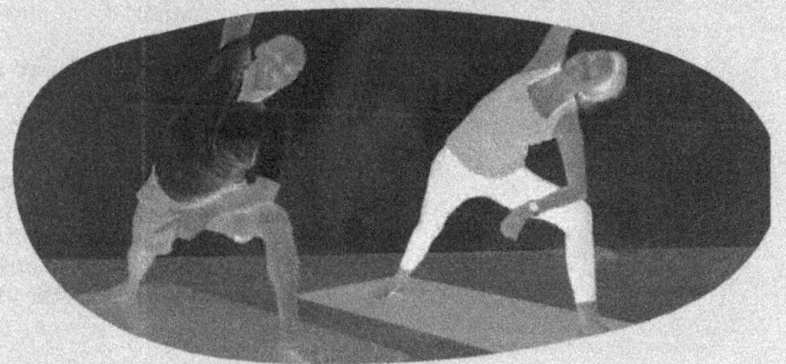

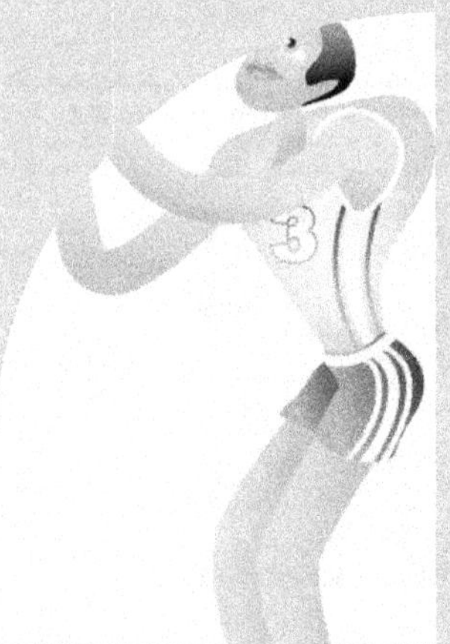

Dynamic Practice

Importance: Engaging in sports like basketball or running integrates physical fitness with mental discipline.

Meaning: These activities emphasize the connection between physical and mental agility, promoting overall well-being.

Practical Application: Incorporate basketball drills or a short run to elevate your heart rate. Use these activities as a form of moving meditation, focusing on your breath and the rhythm of your movements.

Afternoon Routine

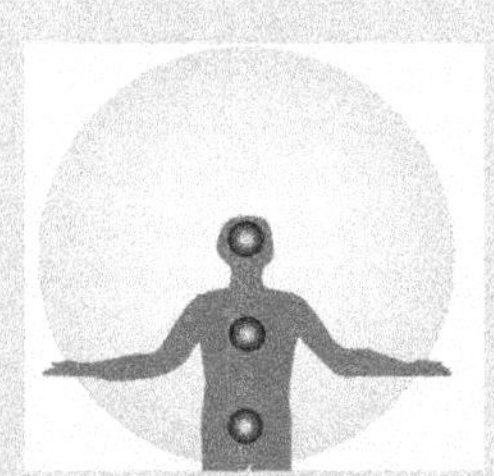

1. 1-15 Minute Flow:

- Take a short break to perform a quick yoga flow.
- Include poses like Cat-Cow, Forward Fold, and Seated Twist.
- Focus on releasing any tension that has built up during the day.

2. Mindful Notes:

- Write down any thoughts, feelings, or insights that have come up.
- Reflect on your progress and areas for growth.

3. Meditative Pause:

- Take a few minutes to sit quietly and focus on your breath.
- Practice a "pause, wait, and respond" meditation to cultivate patience and mindfulness.

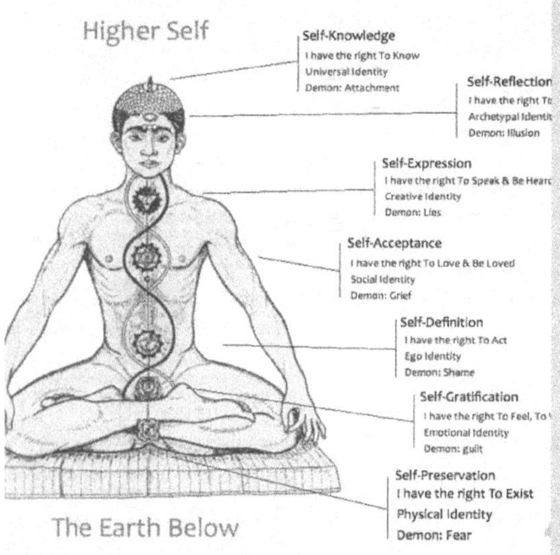

1-15 Minute Flow:

Importance: Short yoga sessions can help to alleviate stress, boost energy, and improve concentration during the day .

Meaning: This quick flow acts as a reset button, helping to maintain focus and productivity.

Practical Application: Take a short break to perform a quick yoga flow. Include poses like Cat-Cow, Forward Fold, and Seated Twist. Focus on releasing any tension that has built up during the day.

Mindful Notes

Importance: Writing down thoughts can enhance self-awareness and emotional processing .

Meaning: This practice encourages reflection and growth, fostering a deeper understanding of oneself.

Practical Application: Write down any thoughts, feelings, or insights that have come up. Reflect on your progress and areas for growth.

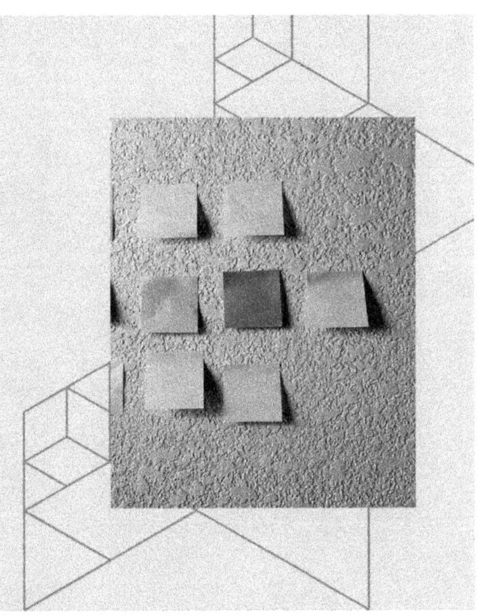

Meditative Pause

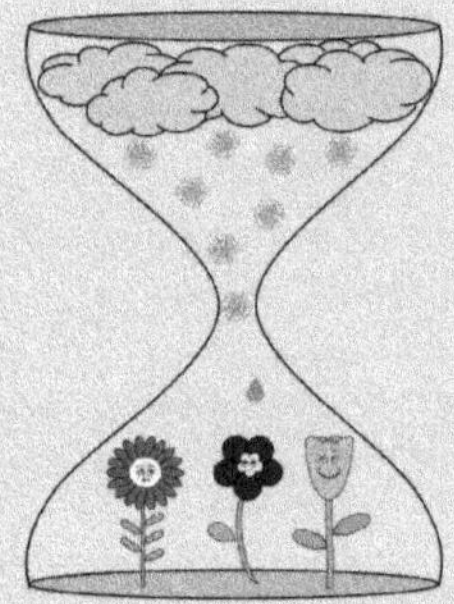

Importance: Brief meditation sessions can reduce stress and anxiety, improving overall mental health .

Meaning: Pausing to meditate cultivates patience and mindfulness, allowing for
thoughtful responses rather than reactions.

Practical Application: Take a few minutes to sit quietly and focus on your breath. Practice a "pause, wait, and respond" meditation to cultivate patience and mindfulness.

Lunch Routine

Mindful Eating:

- Prepare a pescatarian, gluten-free meal.
- Eat slowly and mindfully, savoring each bite.
- Reflect on the source of your food and its journey to your plate.

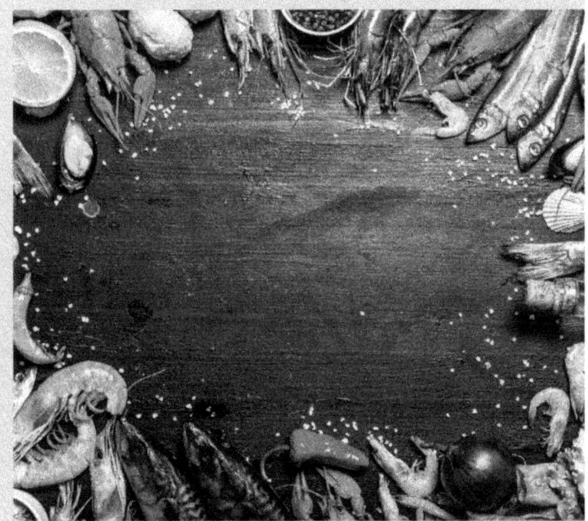

Mindful Eating:

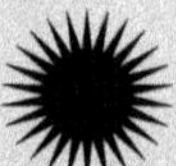 **Importance:** Mindful eating promotes better digestion, prevents overeating, and enhances the enjoyment of food .

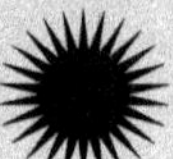 **Meaning:** This practice emphasizes the importance of nourishment and gratitude for the food we consume.

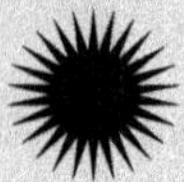 **Practical Application: Prepare a pescatarian,** gluten-free meal. Eat slowly and mindfully, savoring each bite. Reflect on the source of your food and its journey to your plate.

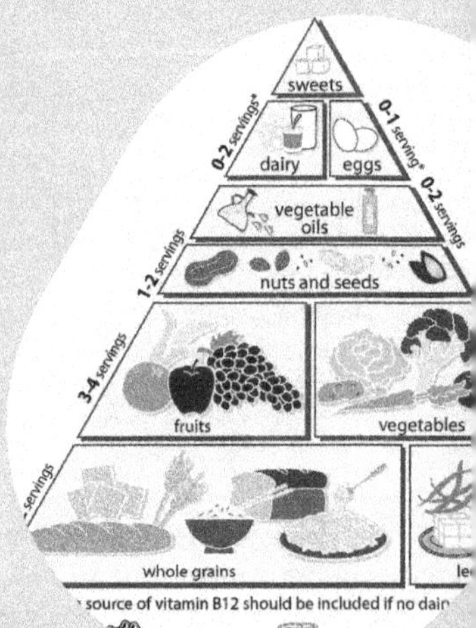

Evening Routine

1. Evening Reflection:
- Spend time reflecting on your day.
- Consider what you have learned and what you are grateful for.

2. Creative Consumption:
- Engage in an activity that stimulates your mind and body, such as reading, drawing, or cooking.

3. Mindful Dinner:
- Eat dinner slowly and mindfully.
- Reflect on the benefits, replicability, and holistic meaning of your food.

4. Yin or Yang Yoga Before Bed:
- Depending on your energy levels and the day's calorie consumption, choose a yin or yang practice.
- Yin Yoga: Focus on deep, restorative poses to relax your body.
- Yang Yoga: Incorporate more dynamic movements to prepare for the next day.

5. One Day at a Time Mantra:
- End your day with the mantra: "One day at a time."
- Acknowledge the importance of best practices and evidence-based living for a healthy life.

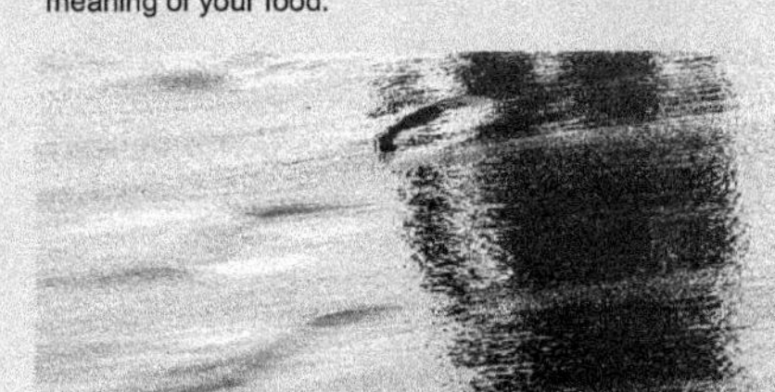

Evening Reflection:

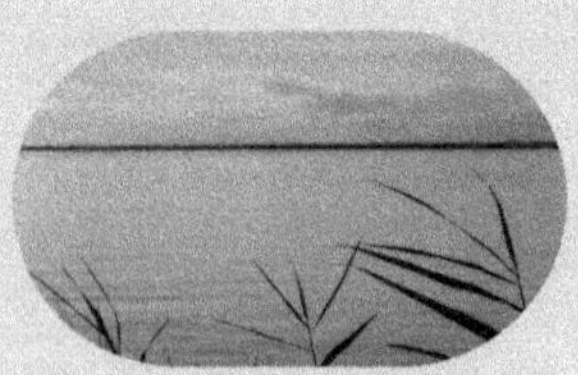

Importance: Reflecting on the day can enhance learning, promote gratitude, and improve sleep quality .

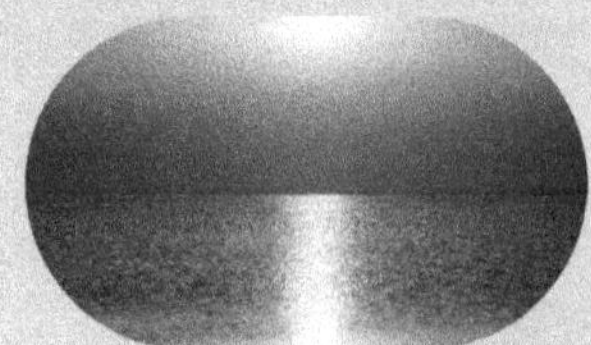

Meaning: This routine encourages mindfulness and appreciation for daily experiences.

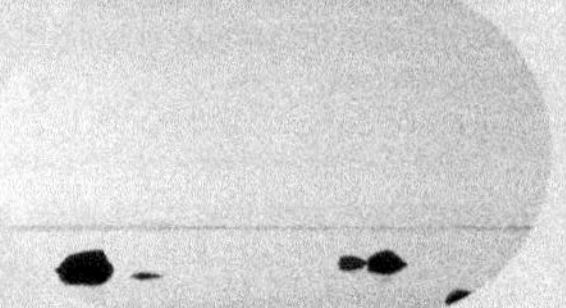

Practical Application: Spend time reflecting on your day. Consider what you have learned and what you are grateful for. Write down any significant insights or moments of gratitude.

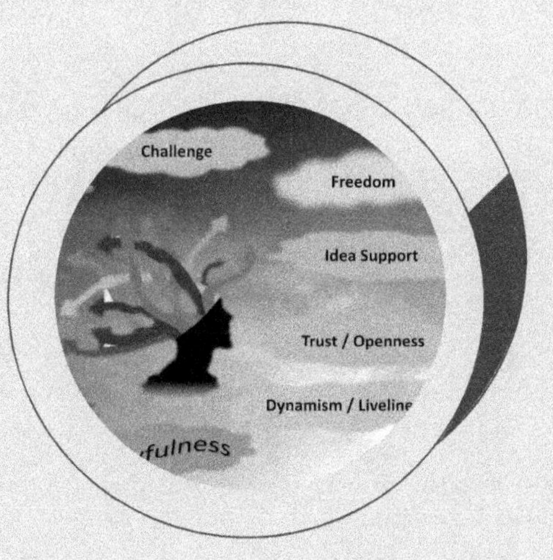

CREATIVE CONSUMPTION:

IMAGINATIVE INTAKE

Importance: Engaging in creative activities stimulates the brain, reduces stress, and fosters personal growth .

Meaning: This practice nurtures creativity and intellectual engagement, enriching the evening experience.

Practical Application: Engage in an activity that stimulates your mind and body, such as reading, drawing, or cooking.

Dinner

Mindful Dinner:

Importance: Eating dinner mindfully can enhance digestion, promote relaxation, and deepen appreciation for food .

Meaning: This routine encourages a holistic view of food, considering its sources, benefits, and impact.

Practical Application: Eat dinner slowly and mindfully. Reflect on the benefits, replicability, and holistic meaning of your food.

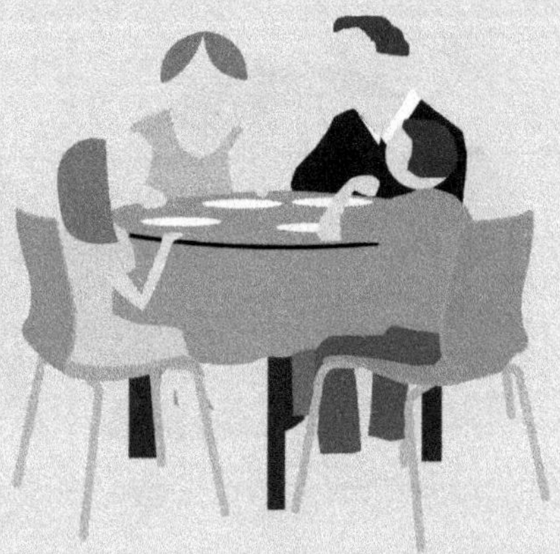

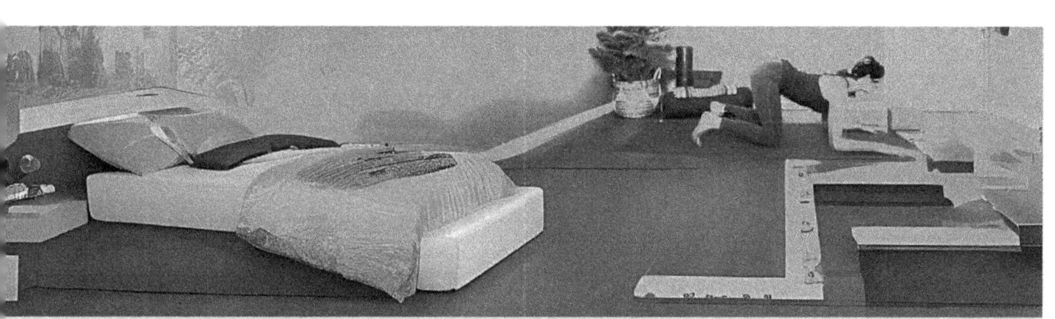

Yin or Yang Yoga Before Bed:

The principles of synergy, where the combined effect is greater than the sum of individual efforts, with the concept of autonomy, highlighting the importance of personal freedom and self-expression within the practice.

Importance: Tailoring evening yoga to energy levels can improve sleep quality and prepare the body for the next day .

Meaning: This practice ensures a balanced approach to physical activity, promoting restful sleep and readiness for tomorrow.

Practical Application: Depending on your energy levels and the day's calorie consumption, choose a yin or yang practice. Yin Yoga: Focus on deep, restorative poses to relax your body. Yang Yoga: Incorporate more dynamic movements to prepare for the next day.

One Day at a Time Mantra:

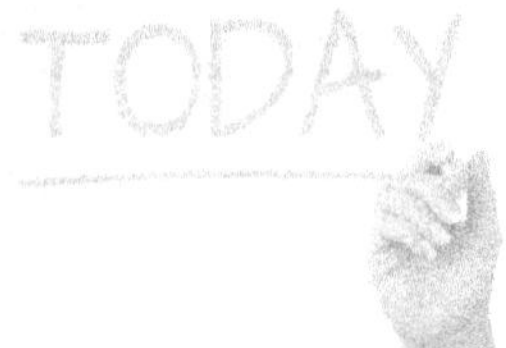

Embrace each dawn's gift ~

Importance: Focusing on the present moment can reduce stress and improve overall well-being .

Meaning: This mantra emphasizes the importance of living mindfully and embracing each day as it comes.

Practical Application: End your day with the mantra: "One day at a time." Acknowledge the importance of best practices and evidence-based living for a healthy life.

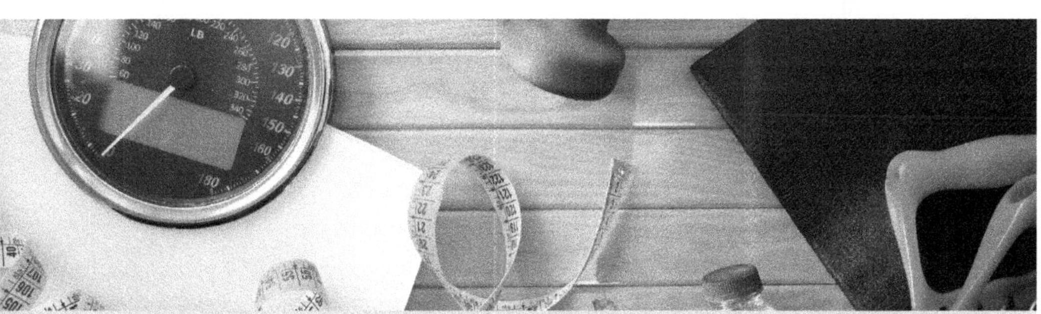

References:

Sources of enchantment

1. Healthline: Benefits of Morning Stretching
2. Harvard Health: The Power of Gratitude
3. WebMD: Benefits of Deep Breathing
4. Mindful: How Mindfulness Changes the Emotional Life of Our Brains
5. Psychology Today: Benefits of Gratitude in Relationships
6. Nature and Health: The Benefits of Outdoor Yoga
7. Verywell Fit: The Benefits of Vinyasa Yoga
8. Mayo Clinic: Exercise and Mental Health
9. American Osteopathic Association: The Benefits of Yoga
10. Psych Central: The Power of Journaling
11. NIH: Meditation for Health
12. Harvard T.H. Chan School of Public Health: The Benefits of Mindful Eating
13. Psychology Today: The Benefits of Reflection
14. Forbes: The Benefits of Creativity
15. Mindful: How Mindful Eating Can Change Your Relationship with Food
16. Sleep Foundation: The Benefits of Yoga for Sleep
17. Mayo Clinic: Stress Management with Mindfulness